Josef Zervas

A manual on the treatment of diseases by electricity employing the faradic current

Josef Zervas

A manual on the treatment of diseases by electricity employing the faradic current

ISBN/EAN: 9783742805805

Manufactured in Europe, USA, Canada, Australia, Japa

Cover: Foto ©Lupo / pixelio.de

Manufactured and distributed by brebook publishing software (www.brebook.com)

Josef Zervas

A manual on the treatment of diseases by electricity employing the faradic current

HISTORICAL.

The use of electricity as a therapeutic agent has been known but a comparatively short time, dating back only one generation. Although since the invention of the electric apparatus, experiments were made to employ the newly discovered force as a therapeutical agent in the treatment of diseases, it was impossible to design and construct an apparatus, fit for medical purposes, until after Faraday's discovery of the electric irritation through the action of magnetic power (1831). The time, when electricity was employed in a scientific manner in the treatment of diseases does not begin until the year 1855, when the work "L' electrisation localisée" was published by the French physician Duchenne. He proved that it was possible to locate the electric current upon certain points beneath the skin, so that every muscle and nerve could be acted upon on any desirable spot.

Since that period, in conjunction with an improved apparatus, a great advance has been made in the use of electricity. Although even at the present time no absolutely clear physical idea exists, what kind of change takes place in the human body, if an organ is affected by the electric current in one way or another, still its actions have been recognized, and it is now well understood, how electricity is to be applied in order to obtain a certain effect.

While at first electric treatment was employed only in affections of the nerves and muscles, paralysis, convulsions, neuralgia, etc., there is, at the present time, hardly any affection, which has not been successfully treated with the electric current. This treatment is denominated: Electro-therapeutic.

The employment of the electric current, as a therapeutical agent, is at the present time confined almost exclusively to physicians and specialists. And it must be admitted, that certain forms of disease on account of the importance of the organs involved, should be treated exclusively by capable specialists, who not only know the importance of the organs affected for the maintenance of life, but are also well versed in the anatomical and pathological branches of the medical science.

In some cases complicated instruments requiring special experience in their application and involving great expense are required, which cannot be successfully employed unless a practical knowledge in handling them has also been gained. However a large number of diseases and especially those occuring most frequently, in the treatment of which electricity is applied, can be successfully treated by any body, who has received proper instruction in the application of the electric current.

Principally three different kinds of electric applications are employed in electro-therapeutics at the present time.

1. The static kind, also called friction electricity or "Franklinism," is generated in the well known manner by means of rotating glass disks and cushions which thus produce the momentary or spark current. This method, however, has been almost entirely abandoned for some time.

2. The "contact electricity" or "Galvanism" is employed in the shape of the constant current. It is generated by certain heterogeneous materials, principally metals, coming in contact with each other, especially if the chemical action of a suitable liquid is brought to bear upon these metals. This apparatus, by means of which this electric current is generated, is generally known under the name of "galvanic battery."

3. Electricity by induction, or Faradism, also known as "Electro-magnetism," has a current, interrupted periodically and at short intervals. It is generated by means of a Rotation apparatus, or, in the same manner of a galvanic current, which latter, however, is systematically divided in single shocks, following each other rapidly. The average price of the cheapest "Rotation apparatus" being as much as the best "Volta Induction Apparatus," because the latter acts automatically, while both the variation of the interrupted current and the regulation of the strength of the current may be extended to

the utmost limits, the latter is without doubt preferable to the "Rotation apparatus," especially as it can be constructed, suitable for transportation in every shape and manner.

Electricity is still employed as a therapeutical agent under different names and in different combinations, yet they must always be reduced to the above mentioned forms, and need, therefore no special mention in this brief essay.

This essay is especially written for the purpose of instructing those who, for some reason or other, are unable or unwilling to avail themselves of the advice of an expert, but are able to keep an electric apparatus of their own. We also believe that even physicians will find some valuable hints in this brief essay, which may induce them to employ electricity more frequently in their private practice. In consequence of this tendency prevailing at the present time, the induction apparatuses are now manufactured more extensively, and comparatively better. They are also cheaper and more practical, than the galvanic batteries with their indispensable additional contrivances. For these reasons it is perfectly proper to treat, with the Faradic current in this essay only.

GENERAL REMARKS.

Of all irritations capable of affecting a nerve, the exciting action of the electric current may be graded with the utmost precision, so that certain well defined symptoms of irritation occur always under similar circumstances and with the utmost regularity. Du Bois Raymond says: the electrical irritation acts on a nerve chiefly at the moment of its beginning and disappearance, also at the moment of its force being suddenly increased or decreased, and, in consequence thereof, principally through the fluctuation of the current, and not through the absolute value of the intensity of the current used at that time, because, the more intensely the nerve is excited, the more suddenly the density of the current increases or decreases on its passing through the nerve. Von

Betzold, Benedict and Wundt add, as a supplement: not only the closing and opening of the current acts in an exciting manner on nerves of motion and sensation, but partially, the constantly acting current too.

Currents of too great strength hinder the conducting capacity through a reduction of the excitability. The electrical stimulation is most effective in longitudinal currents, it becomes ineffective if applied vertically to the nerve axis. The muscle twitches soonest, if the current passes in a transverse direction. (Sachs.) If the current is passed in a longitudinal direction, the exciting action increases, if the current remains the same in strength, in proportion to the length of the tract through which the current passes, and, the farther remote from the muscle the positive pole and, the nearer to it, the negative pole is applied, the stronger is the effect obtained with the same strength of the currents. (Hermann, Willy.) The excitability of the nerves of motion is greater than that of the muscular tissue if deprived of their nerves of sensation. The nerves of the flexor muscles are easier excited than those of the extensor muscles. The same rule applies to the flexor and extensor muscles.

The normal excitability of the nerves is proportionate to their normal nutrition. If the latter is wanting, a higher excitability of the nerves is first observed, but after the nerve is materially injured, diminution occurs. Hence the increase of excitability means a reduction of nerve power (sive energy). Continued excitement of the nerves and also exertion of the muscles, without any intermediate rest, cause at first fatigue and exhaustion, and finally excitability decreases sufficiently, until lost completely. A continued inaction is also followed by the same results as overexertion. (Dr. R. Lewandowski.) Recovery takes place sooner in the nerves, than in the muscles.

SPECIAL.

The sanative actions of inducted currents are, like in galvanism, of an (*a*) exciting, (*b*) modifying and (*c*) catalytic nature.

Dry metallic electrodes are used for the purpose of acting upon the skin, while electrodes, having a wet sponge or cover attached, are used for influencing the subcutaneous tissues.

a. In order to obtain an exciting effect upon the surface of the body, the brush electrode is employed, (the other electrode may be of any available kind, provided the electrode has a wet sponge or cover attached to it, when held steadily). The brush is then either moved over the skin, or it is applied to it and then taken off, or, it is kept closely to the skin without touching it, when sparks are seen to leap over to the skin.

The nerves may be best excited, if isolated, by an application to their motor points. The muscles may be excited either directly, or indirectly, by exciting the motor nerve, whereby clonic as well as tetanic contractions are obtained. It is possible to affect through reflex action, even more deeply situated tissues, by applying the brush to the skin.

If it is intended to directly affect the natural cavities of the body (pharynx, stomach, intestines, urethra, bladder, uterus), lined by mucous membranes and easy of access, the Faradic will be found more appropriate than the galvanic current, because the latter may, through electrolysis (chemical decomposition) cauterize the mucous membrane wherever it is applied.

The production of clonic muscular contractions improves nutrition by stimulating the flow of the secretions, it also induces, as it were, a sort of gymnastic exercise, whereby the inactive muscles may be preserved against secondary degeneration. Debilitated, antagonizing muscles are also strengthened wherever there is an affection of the muscles, sinews and joints, for instance in stiffness from inactivity and paralysis (paresis) following fractures, dislocations, resections, ligatures applied for a long period, also in inflammation of the sheaths of tendons and pseudarthrosis (false joints). Organs in which the smooth muscular fibre prevails, are also stimulated to normal action (stomach, intestines, reduction of incarcerated hernia, bladder, uterus). Glandular organs are also made to contract and evacuate their contents, their volume is also diminished in a lasting manner, even if Faradisation has been suspended (as in paralysis of the bladder, enuresis—sive incontinence of urine, nocturnal spermatorrhoe—sive flow of semen, increased labor pains, as a styptic, the removal of amenorhoe and dysmenorrhoe, abnormal position of the uterus and contraction of the spleen).

Tonic muscular contractions of the diaphragm, through Faradic stimulation of the phrenic nerves are used for the induction of artificial respiration, in asphyxia, caused by the inhalation of carbonic acid, gas, etc., excessive use of opium or alcohol, diphtheria. The stimulation of the phrenicus is caused by applying both poles, thoroughly wet, simultaneously to both phrenic nerves, or by placing one pole upon the phrenic nerve and the other on the pit of the stomach. The current is interrupted every two to three seconds, for an equal period, in order to excite rhythmic respiration. Singultus is treated in a similar way, yet without interruption of the current.

b. The modifying actions of the Faradic current do not depend upon the actions of the poles, as in the galvanic current, for they also are merely stimulating. They resemble, however, in their effect the modifying actions of the galvanic current. The application of the Faradic brush produces, both a continued increase of the sensitiveness of the skin, and also a reduction of the sense of pain in the skin. For this reason the application of the Faradic brush for removing anaesthesia (insensibility), as an actual stimulus to the skin, is better than any other remedy, while the application of the moistened electrode removes all pain. This kind of application has been successful in temporary relaxation of paralytic contraction and hemiplegia (one sided paralysis and curvature), while Duchenne attempted to stretch contracted muscles through Faradisation of the antagonizing (counter) muscle. Weak Faradic currents animate the excitability of the nerves, strong currents, however, reduce excitability. The application of the brush to the skin, chest, arms and back, with a current of medium strength of five to six minutes duration, produces a contraction of the cerebral vessels and also cerebral anaemia. A weak peripheral application hastens the circulation of the blood, together with an increased action of the heart and contracts the caliber of the blood vessels. Strong currents produce the opposite effect. An energetic Faradic brushing of the skin diminishes the flow of blood towards the deeply situated organs, by causing hyperaemia of the skin. It thus becomes, both a powerful derivative and revulsive means (derivation and distribution of the liquids contained in the human body). The treatment of tubercular as well as other chronic affections of the spinal marrow turns upon those facts.

c. The catalytic (dissolving) action of the Faradic current has been established through the numerous practical results obtained therefrom. They are produced both by the application of the brush as well as through the employment of moist electrodes. To this category belong, also, the resorbing actions of the Faradic current in lumbago, inflammatory rheumatism of the joints, dropsy, enlargement of the lymphatic glands, etc.

Before proceeding to consider the single pathological symptoms, we cannot but quote from the writing of Dr. *Carl* Neumann, the most important parts as given by him briefly and in a superior manner.

I. The irritation of a muscles, which is evidently necessary for curing paralytic conditions, may be accomplished *directly*, by placing the thoroughly moistened electrodes, close to each other upon the paralytic muscle.

II. The irritation of the muscle happens in an *indirect* manner, if the nerve, belonging to the muscle is irritated.

III. The irritation of the muscle may be divided by applying one electrode to the muscle, and the other to the nerve belonging to the muscle.

IV. The direct irritation of the muscle implies the use of a stronger current, than the indirect irritation.

V. The indirect irritation of a muscle is not possible to such an extent as, direct irritation, sometimes it is even inert, if the nerve belonging to the muscle enters the deep portion.

VI. Faradisation of a muscle stimulates this muscle in an artificial manner, into increased activity and, consequently promotes the circulation of the blood, and the excretion of effective matter, and regulates the condition of the temperature.

VII. A succession of feeble Faradisations, not strong enough to cause muscular twitchings, increases the irritability sufficiently, to cause finally muscular twitchings. Faradisation has consequently an animating quality.

VIII. It is possible, in consequence of this animating property of the inducted current, to stop the atrophic degeneration of the muscular tissue, and to strengthen the muscle anew.

IX. The inducted current, also, causes a dilatation of the bloodvessel, thus removing any stagnation of the blood current.

X. The inducted current has therefore an antiphlogistic influence.

XI. Faradisation may also promote the flow of liquids within the human body (between the two electrodes), i. e. it produces a so-called cataphoric action.

XII. Faradisation has frequently been employed successfully, decomposing liquids in an electric manner, i. e. the so-called electrolysis.

XIII. The catalytic phenomena just mentioned, has as a final result the resorption of morbidly excreted matter.

XIV. The inducted current is especially important as a stimulant to the skin. This stimulation of the skin, produced through the application of the electrical brush, assists in the removal of interrupted sensation, while a tonic influence is brought to bear upon the diseased brain in cases of paralysis.

XV. . The inducted current is a powerful anodyne in so-called Neuralgias, which affection is supposed to mean an affection of the sheaths and of the manner of the sensor nerves.

XVI. Faradisation of the entire body, in which every part of it is exposed to the action of the current, is very useful in certain cases and, frequently its effect is equal to that of static electricity.

XVII. In treating very sensitive patients for an affection of the face, the best method would be the *electric hand*, that is, the patient grasps one electrode (the negative pole) with his hand, while the physician (or some other person) holds in his hand the other electrode (the positive pole), while the other hand or a single finger, after being moistened, is passed over the affected parts. Instead of direct touching with the hand or finger, a small moistened sponge may be used in the same manner.

XVIII. If the skin alone is to be treated, it is best to render it a bad conductor, i. e. it must be in a thoroughly dried condition, which is easily attained by covering it with a layer of powdered chalk.

THE FARADIC APPARATUS AND THE ELECTRODES.

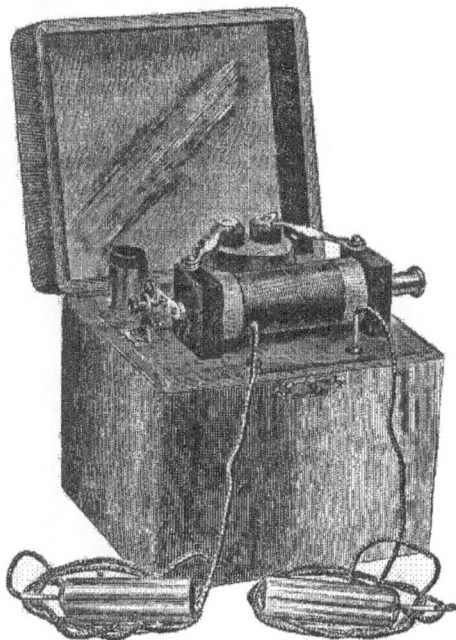

In addition to the apparatus there will also be furnished :

a. Two plain cylindric Metallic Electrodes with universal handles, to be used as hand and dry electrodes, or as foot and stable electrodes in general Faradisation, as well as immersion in the electric bath.

These dry electrodes can easily be changed into moist electrodes by pressing one half of a suitable piece of sponge firmly into the mouth of the cylinder while the other or outer half forms the pole to be applied.

b. The roller electrode which consists of a carbon cylinder

covered with a coat of felt, is to be used as a moist electrode, to be applied steadily to one spot and, also, for the purpose of passing it over large portions of the body.

    c. The brush or pencil-electrode for stimulating the skin. See special points, (*a*) irritative effects.

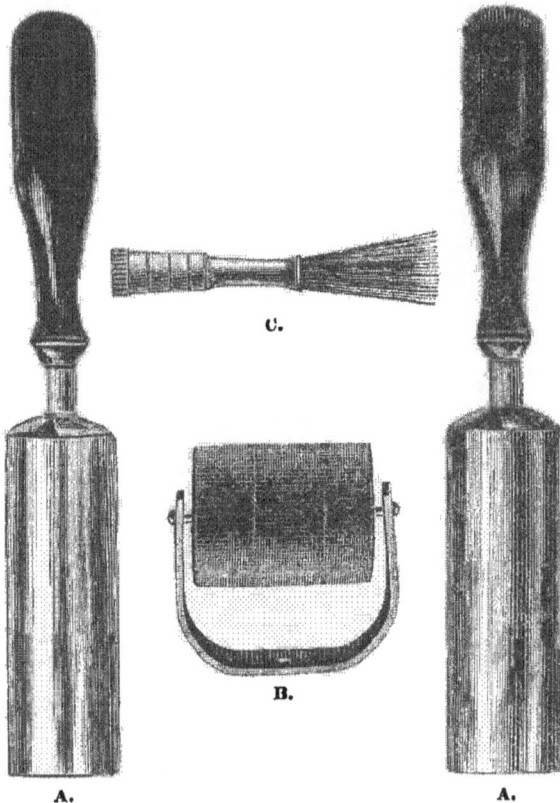

CUTS SHOWING ELECTRODES.

It remains for us to give a few well proved directions concerning the simple application of Faradisation, not yet mentioned in this essay.

    General Faradisation is as follows : the Kathode (the negative pole) is applied, as the largest possible electrode, to the feet or nates, while the Anode (the positive pole) is gradually passed over the entire surface of the body. For this manipulation the moistened roller electrode is to be used. A simple, warm foot bath in which the negative pole is immersed will serve best as a foot-electrode. If the patient's feet are too sensitive, a wet sponge had better be attached to the negative pole, before being applied to the nates. The order most in use for passing the roller electrode over the body is as follows: the neck, especially on both sides of the vertebral column, for about two minutes, the entire muscular system of the back for about three minutes, the muscles of the chest and abdomen three to four minutes, the upper and lower extremities for one to two minutes. Finally the head by means of the electric hand, one to two minutes. The term *electric hand* has already been explained on page 10, paragraph XVII.

The *electric hand* is to be used in Faradisation of the face, of the organs of sense or, of the head.

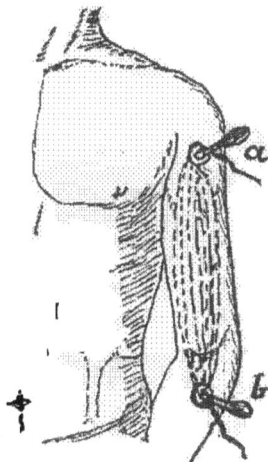

FIGURE 1.

Figure 1 is a sketch, showing how electricity passes through the body. *A* and *b* are the two electrodes. The current enters the body at *a*, *b* being the point of exit. We are not to imagine that the electrical current represents, as it were, a compact thread, but rather a filiform bundle of an indefinite number of threads, which branch out from the point of entrance, and re-unite at the point of exit, always bent upon however, to pass in the shortest possible route between the two terminal points. The intensity of the current will therefore be greatest and at the same time strongest, at the two points *a* and *b*. The current will, however, act upon the entire tract in proportion to its strength, density and duration. The poorest conductors on the body are the hair, nails and callosities of the skin. A dry skin is a worse conductor than a moist one. The bones also, are poorer conductors than the muscular tissue. The Faradic current overcomes resistance far easier than the galvanic current. The former is also felt less unpleasant than the latter. The positive pole is easily distinguished, by the touch, from the negative pole, because the latter which may be considered as the pole of entrance, causes a stronger effect than the former.

If the seat of an illness is known, the local electric treatment is the best. If unknown, the entire system in which the affected spot is supposed to be, must be cautiously subjected to the electrical treatment.

In commencing the electrical treatment it is best to employ a weak current at first and increase it gradually. They must not, however, cause an irksome, but rather a pleasant sensation. By the scale attached to the sliding cylinder of the induction apparatus, the operator will easily be able to ascertain, in a sufficiently exact manner the suitable strength of the current for further treatment. If it is, however, doubtful which side of the body is affected, comparative experiments will soon indicate which side is to be treated, because man is shaped in a pre-eminently symmetrical manner.

The duration of an electric session depends of course, upon the nature of the affection, and the patient's constitution. Sensitive persons require a shorter time than those of a more robust nature. As a rule, the duration of the treatment will vary from one and a half to ten minutes. One application daily, or every two or three days will be sufficient. However a certain regularity ought to be observed. It has been found advantageous to suspend the electric treatment for a period of from one to two weeks, after it has been continued for one to two months.

As we do not intend to write a general learned essay but, rather a common place review and also, a practical instruction for the non-professional operator, how to employ Faradic electricity in certain cases, we may now be allowed to mention the special cases of illness in which the use of electricity is recommended.

We have carefully chosen, the latest and most approved methods of renowned specialists, and whatever our own experience has taught us, those methods which we have found to be the easiest and most simple ones for our purpose.

As the patient, in many cases will be able to apply the electrical treatment himself, a detrimental and excessive application of a too powerful current will be prevented as a rule.

However, we emphatically repeat, that the proper application of the current, and not its strength, is instrumental in curing disease. If the treatment is in other hands, it is advisable to begin with a weak current, gradually increasing its strength, until the suitable degree of strength is attained for each individual case.

DISEASES AND THEIR TREATMENT.

Agoraphobia—Horror Vacui. This peculiar nervous condition shows itself in a general feeling of anxiety, fits of alarm, together with an idea of a possible accident, it also attacks the patient while walking about the streets or public places, traveling in dazzling sunshine, being crowded by a multitude of people, fear if left in small rooms with a low ceiling, etc.

Treatment: General Faradisation by means of electric bath, a temperature of 90—95° F., with one electrode immersed in the bath while the other is applied to the neck or to any other part of the body not covered by the water. In holding the second electrode in the hand, it is advisable to change it every two to three minutes from one hand to the other.

Duration of bath up to twenty minutes, one bath to be taken every one to two days.

Agrypnia—sleeplessness, as a consequence of a general affection or of local disease. Treatment: General Faradisation has been successful.

Amaurosis—blindness and *Amblyopia—weakened eye-sight,* from inflammation and atrophy of the nerves of sight.

Treatment consists of applying the Faradic brush to the back, or, with a weak current, the positive pole is applied to the brow, the negative pole to the neck. Duration two to five minutes daily.

Amenorrhoea—absence of the menses. Treatment : The positive pole is applied to the loins, and the negative pole to the lower part of the abdomen, and a moderate current is brought to bear upon it about ten minutes, shortly before the regular time for the appearance of the monthly sickness.

Anaemia—poverty of the blood.

a. *Of the brain.* This condition may be caused by various circumstances such as, copious bleeding, long continued fever, convulsions, deficient nourishment, chronic diarrhœa, excessively long nursing of children.

Treatment: Depends upon the primary cause, see the remarks below, also convulsions, etc.

b. *Pernicious anaemia*, deficiency of red corpuscles. Patients suffering from this dangerous affection, gradually assume a pale yellow-tinged appearance and complain of great debility, dyspnœa, palpitation of the heart and from the slightest movement, a feeling of fullness at the pit of the stomach often accompanied by vomiting. Next follow bleeding from the nose, effusion of blood under the skin and frequently a high degree of fever. These symptoms are generally caused by malnutrition, excessive bodily and mental exertion, too frequent confinements, prolonged nursing of children and every other symptom mentioned for anaemia of the brain.

Treatment: General electrization, to be continued for some time, in order to act upon the entire suffering nervous system, has really produced many wonderful cures in such cases. It is of course necessary to enjoin in these as well as in other diseases, a proper mode of living and a suitable diet with plenty of fresh air.

Anaesthesia—insensibility, especially of the *skin* and *muscles.* Causes : Division and impaired nutrition of the nerves, chronic metallic poisoning, ligation of blood vessels, pressure by tumors etc., upon the nerves and disease of the bones. Frequently there exists still the local sensation of pressure and temperature, while only the feeling of pain has entirely disappeared. This is called "Analgesia." Also the mucous membranes may become anaesthetic, i. e. insensible to pain.

Treatment: The Faradic brush is applied to the skin by passing, with a powerful current, the negative pole over the affected part daily for about ten minutes, while the positive pole is placed upon the spinal roots of the back bone.

Angina pectoris, stenocardia—spasm of the heart, which mostly attacks persons living in damp, cold rooms, suffering from colds and given to excessive tobacco smoking. It is recognized by a painful sensation of constriction, together with a feeling of great anxiety, beginning over the region of the heart and mostly extending over the left side of the body. There is also palpitation of the heart, an irregular pulse, paleness of the face, cold hands and feet, and a cold clammy skin.

Treatment: Strong Faradisation around the nipples, and general Faradisation in the electric bath, and application of the negative pole to the cervical portion of the spinal column.

Angioparalysis—vascular paralysis; occurs especially in hysterical persons with weak nerves. It is accompanied by a quick pulse, palpitation of the heart, dizziness, scintillation before the eyes, headache, redness of the skin with increase of its temperature. If these symptoms are restricted to the fingers and toes only, it is called "Erythromelalgia."

Treatment: Application of the Faradic brush or, of the moistened electrode upon the affected part.

Anidrosis, or *deficient perspiration*, or inertness of the sweat glands are treated in a like manner.

It is a peculiar fact that the effect of the direct electrical treatment of the entire system of nerves, in one way or another may be of a manifold and most peculiar character (Dr. C. Neumann).

Anidrosis—inability of the skin to perspire. Treatment: General Faradisation or electric baths.

Aphony—paralysis of the vocal cords is, a paralysis of the laryngeal nerves, the seat of which may be either central or peripheral.

Treatment: The positive pole is placed upon the neck, while the Faradic brush is passed for three to four minutes over the external laryngeal region.

Arthritis deformans—knotted gout of the joints. Occurs fre-quently after rheumatism of joints, especially of the hip and of the lesser joints.

Treatment: Electrical baths with moistened electrodes and brush which are applied to both sides of the joint, so that the most intense current may pass through. The baths, either as full baths of the entire body, or of the affected joints alone, should be taken several times during the day, for the period of one quarter to one half hour if great pain exists, while be-tween times local Faradisation may also be used. Excellent results have been obtained by this method.

Asphyxia—apparent death, paralysis of the organs of respira-tion, see page 7, Article *a*: stimulating effects.

Asthma—difficult respiration. Treatment: General Farad-isation. It has been of great success, applying both poles for one quarter to one half an hour, twice a day, to the region of the thyroid cartilage or to the angle of the jaw bone. Also application of the Faradic brush to the region of the heart and the nipple.

Atonia—relaxation of the stomachic and intestinal muscles, dilatation of the stomach. Treatment: The negative pole is applied to the region of the stomach, the positive pole about to the region of the third thoracic spondyle. With a strong current lasting for about four minutes, the negative pole is passed gently over the region of the stomach.

Cardialgia—Gastrodynia. Neuralgia of the stomach, cramps of the stomach, is an affection of the nervus vagus, and also of that part of the sympathetic nerve, supplying the stomach.

Treatment: Faradic brush applied to the region over the heart and to the nipple, also the application of one pole over the pit of the stomach, and of the other upon the spinal column. Daily two to three times, from five to ten minutes.

Catalepsy, see Eclipsis.

Cerebral apoplexy or *Apoplexia cerebri* means an effusion of blood from a broken cerebral bloodvessel into the substance of the brain.

Treatment: The electrical current is useless until some four to five weeks after the attack. In the meantime the treatment in use in such cases will be of advantage, viz.:

rest and cold application to the head. After this period electrical treatment is advisable. The positive pole is placed upon the neck behind the ascending portion of the inferior maxillary bone, while the negative pole is applied to the opposite side, close to the cervical column, as nearly as possible between the cervical vertebra, and the eighth vertebra. A very weak current is then allowed to pass through this part for about one, to one and a half minutes. Electrization of any possibly paralyzed portion of the body must also be applied, alternating with the application just mentioned, according to the rules adopted in cases of paralysis. On the whole, the galvanic treatment has been tried more frequently in cases of apoplexy.

Chilblains. Treatment: One or both feet are placed in an electrical foot bath. One electrode is applied to the swelling with a powerful current for about ten to fifteen minutes duration daily, the other electrode is place in the bath.

Chlorosis—poverty of blood. (Deficiency of red blood corpuscles in the female.)

Treatment: General Faradisation every other day has been successful in many cases. Others, caused by mechanical disturbances, such as curvature of the spine, were cured by the author of this essay, through an invention of the author, " the Health Restorer Belt."

Chorea—St. Vitus' Dance. Symptoms: Involuntary spasmodic motions of single muscles, or groups of muscles, beyond the control of the individual will.

Treatment: General Faradisation, one to two times daily, has a favorable influence, also passing one pole over the spinal column, chest and abdomen, while the patient takes the other pole into his hands.

Chronic Inflammation of the Joints. Treatment: The affected joints are exposed to the action of the Faradic current for about ten minutes. This is to be continued daily until the patient is cured. See also under " Treatment of Arthritis."

Cystitis Catarrhales—Catarrh of the Bladder, and Cystospasmus—Spasm of the Bladder. Treatment: The negative pole is applied with its largest surface to the region of the bladder next to the symphysis pubis, while the positive pole is passed gently over the lower portion of the cervical column, and the sacral region on either side from above downwards for about three to four minutes.

Dysmenorrhœa—Painful Menstruation. Treatment: The same as in amenorrhœa.

Dyspepsia—Nervous disturbance of digestion. Treatment: General Faradisation and electrical baths. Also the Faradic current is applied, with the largest possible surface and proceeding from the two hips transversely across the abdomen. The latter method has been followed by brilliant results.

Eclipsis—Catalepsy. Is a suddenly occurring stiffness of the muscular system, whereby the body remains in exactly the same position in which it happened to be, at the beginning of the attack.

Treatment: General Faradisation.

*Enuresis nocturna—*Incontinence of urine during the night. Treatment: The same as in cystitis. In children, however, the current must be very weak.

Epilepsy, Morbus sacer. Epileptic Fit. Treatment: General Faradisation is recommended once daily, also electrical baths every two days.

Erysipelas—King's evil. Treatment: The affected part is covered with a layer of solution of iodide of potash, or, if not on hand, with cloths dipped in salt or ammonia water, over these Faradisation is applied daily for about ten minutes. Swellings and affections of a similar kind are treated in the same manner.

Gangrene. Treatment: General Faradisation, especially of the stomach, heart, lungs and spinal column twice daily.

*Gastrodynia—*Cramps of the stomach, see Cardialgia.

Graphospasmus— Writer's cramps is a spasm of the extensor or flexor muscles of the fingers, mostly of the latter. In this affection the thumb is bent inwards, and the hand and the forearm quiver spasmodically.

Treatment: Faradisation of the affected muscles with moist electrodes, feeble at first, moderately increased to a medium strength.

If the extensor muscles of the forearm are affected, the

electrical treatment must be directed to the radial nerves and the muscles supplied by the nerves; if the flexor muscles are to be treated, the medium ulnar nerves and the muscles under its control are to be Faradised. Every other similar spasmodic symptom is to be treated in a similar manner.

Headache. Pain of the head, nervous or from some other cause, pressure on the head, also a feeling of heaviness and desolation in the same, sleeplessness, ill temper approaching melancholy, are successfully improved and even cured through the application of a *weak* Faradic current, both with the moistened roller electrode, and especially with the electric hand. The patient takes one electrode in his hand, or if an assistant is on hand, in both hands, then the current is applied with the roller, or the electrical hand from the neck around to the forehead, for about five minutes. It is more difficult to subdue a violent attack, than to cure the affection entirely by daily electrization, continued for some length of time between the several attacks.

Other similar symptoms, requiring however a different treatment, are described elsewhere under the proper headings.

Hemicrania. Sick headache is an affection of the sympathetic nerve, attacks mostly women, generally every four weeks, at the beginning of the monthly sickness. The causes of this troublesome, though not dangerous illness are: Excessive mental exertion, immoderate indulgence in strong coffee, tea, spirituous liquors, also inherited, etc. Symptoms are: An ill temper, yawning, chilliness, headache with great sensitiveness to sounds and bright light, and sickness of the stomach.

Treatment: Faradisation of the painful spot with the electrical hand, (see page 10) from three to four minutes with a current of medium power.

Hyperidrosis—Profuse perspiration. If this is merely a symptom of some diseases which are accompanied by fever, an accelerated action of the heart and an increased pressure of the blood in the vascular system, electrical treatment is not advisable. But if the above mentioned affection is followed by a chronic increased perspiration, general electrization will then prove successful, frequently even after a short time.

Hypochondria is a proper subject for electrical treatment only, for the alleviation of certain symptoms (constipation, disturbance of the sexual organs, insomnolency, pressure on the head, a feeling of distress etc.), treatment on general principles (as in debility of the nerves). Whenever the cause of these complaints can be ascertained, general electrization, with a weak current is advisable.

Hysteria. Treatment: General Faradisation with a medium current and electrical baths have been followed by excellent results.

Impotence—Debility of the sexual organs. Treatment: In addition to the stimulating action of the electrical bath, the Faradic brush may also be used. One pole is applied to the loin, while the other, with brush attached, is passed over the perineal and rectal region for three to four minutes. When this is done, the brush is passed thirty to forty times over either spermatic cord, as well as over the upper and lower surface of the penis.

Ischias—Pain of the sciatic nerve. Treatment: One electrode, with the broadest possible surface is placed as the positive pole upon the point of exit of the sciatic nerve, while the brush, as the negative pole, is passed every one to two days, for about ten minutes, along the sciatic tract as far as the pain extends. It would be well to frequently include the os sacrum also. For the negative pole an electrical foot bath may be used, by putting one foot into the bath, the positive pole being arranged as mentioned before. A similar treatment is recommended in:

Ischias antica or crural neuralgia, sive—Ischiadia passion (neuralgia of the thigh). Treatment applied to the muscles supplied by the nerve just mentioned.

Ischury—Paralysis of the bladder. Treatment: One electrode is applied to the symphysis of the pubic bone, and the other to the perineum for about four minutes. Alternating with this the spinal marrow is Faradised, with a weak current for two to three minutes.

Mastodynia—Neuralgia of the mammary gland. Is ushered

in with violent pain, proceeding from the mammary gland to the shoulder, arm and back, sometimes it is accompanied by vomiting. Girls at the age of puberty are principally affected, the pain increasing at the monthly period. This affection is quite obstinate.

Treatment: Daily application of the Faradic brush to the corresponding side of the breast and back for about five to ten minutes with a current of moderate strength.

Megrim—Sick headache. See Hemicrania.

Menorrhagia—Profuse menstruation. Treatment: Vigorous Faradisation of the lower abdominal region with the negative pole, while the positive pole is applied to the loins.

Morbus Basedowii is principally observed in the female sex, it is accompanied by rapid palpitation of the heart (with a pulse of one hundred and twenty to one hundred and forty a minute), enlargement of the thymus gland (goitre), protrusion of the eyes (staring eyes). Disturbance of the monthly period, neuralgia, etc., have also been observed.

Treatment: General electrization and electric baths every other day, to be continued for some time. Also Faradisation of the sympathetic nerve in the meantime.

Nervous Vomiting. Treatment: Faradisation from the back or neck to the epigastric region (upper abnominal region), for about three to five minutes daily.

Neuralgia. A painful affection of the nerves, is a violent pain, attacking the nerves of sensation from time to time, often occuring from slight causes. Pressure upon the trunk of the nerve may alleviate the pain. There are, naturally, a variety of neuralgic pains, some kinds of which we have already described under the proper heading.

There remains, however, to be mentioued an especial affection, viz. :

a. Neuralgia of the fifth nerve, also called *Tic douloureux.* This affection generally attacks the nerve of one side only, along the track of the Trigeminus (see Figure). Its three most important branches supply the eyes, the upper and lower jaw bone, then branching out in many directions.

Treatment: General Faradisation, also the application of

the brush to the painful spot, with the other electrode resting upon the neck. May be repeated several times daily.

b. Cervico-occipital Neuralgia. Neuralgia of the neck and posterior portion of the head is treated by general Faradisation, and also, by applying the moist electrodes directly to the affected spot.

c. Neuralgia lumbo-abdominalis. Neuralgia of the lumbar vertebrae, is treated by passing the Faradic brush over the lower portion of the back, nates, abdominal wall and loins for about ten minutes each time.

d. Intercostal neuralgia. Neuralgic intercostal pain. Requires application of Faradic brush. The same treatment will do for every other kind of neuralgia.

Neurasthenia. General debility of the nervous system; is met with more frequently in men than in women. This is an affection of the sympathetic nerves and their branches, accompanied by irritation of the brain and spinal marrow, a malady differing from hypochondriasis and hysteria. The following symptoms are observed : Rapid exhaustion of the entire system of muscles and nerves, hyperaesthesia, easy excitability, abdominal complaints, debility of the lungs and heart, asthma, anguish of the heart, relaxation, weakness of the organs of sense, chronic catarrh of the nose, excessive perspiration, etc.

Treatment: General Faradisation, also the Faradic brush with a mild current are followed by very favorable results.

Obesitas—Obesity. Treatment the same as in dyspepsia.

Obstructio alvi. Constipation is removed by vigorous Faradisation of the abdominal muscles daily, from two to three times for about fifteen minutes. Also

Occlusion of the large intestine. Same treatment.

Paresis. Incomplete paralysis and *paralysis* caused by apoplexy (central).

The application of electricity, in this affection, is the best remedial agent known. We shall mention this subject somewhat more in detail as the remarks here made shall also convey general, useful hints concerning the diagnosis and treatment of other pathological symptoms. Electrical treatment will be useful both in paresis and paralysis, not only in that part of the central system of nerves from which the trunks of the nerves supplying the paralyzed muscles are derived, but also those in which are situated the nutrition centres of the ailing portion of the body. In these cases the paralyzed nerve trunks are directly influenced through the stimulating action of the electrical current, improving circulation and nutrition, and also, by increasing the irritability of the nerves, the disturbances in the system, following the above mentioned affections are obviated. Furthermore, the resorbing action of the electrical current, removes the disturbances caused by the seat of the disease.

For the purpose of obtaining reflex actions, it will be best to select the shortest reflex arc; for instance, in facial paralysis of the trigeminus nerve, in spinal paralysis the corresponding nerves of sense and spinal roots. Irritation of the skin will bring on vaso-motor * changes in the central nerve organs, functional disturbances will also influence in the same way ; thus Faradisation of the skin will improve the power of speaking. For the same purpose Faradisation of the nerves of motion with moist electrodes will be found useful. The application of the Faradic brush to certain parts of the skin from one to two square inches in size, for fifteen to thirty minutes, wherever paralysis exists, will likewise answer the purpose. The Faradic brushing of more extended portions of the skin of the back and extremities with the negative pole of the inducted current, while the moistened positive pole is placed upon the sternum (breast bone). The use of a weak current for a longer period is better borne than that of a more powerful one for a shorter period. If it is intended to bring a general influence to bear upon the entire body, general Faradisation with the roller electrode, or the electrical bath is to be preferred. The length of time and the particular kind of electrical treatment is to be adapted to the patient and also, to the situation, eventually also by actual experiment.

Pollutions and Spermatorrhoea. Involuntary effusion of semen is treated in the same manner as cystitis. The penis

---

* Sympathetic or ganglia-system of nerves, which seems to be merely to cause activity in the vessels.

and perineum are also to be taken into consideration, if necessary, in which case the positive pole remains firmly placed upon the lumbar region.

Rheumatism. Faradisation has been successful in almost every kind of rheumatic affection (muscular, acute and chronic, also rheumatism of the joints), both with the application of the moist electrodes as also, of the Faradic brush, or a combination of both. The poles are always to be placed in such a manner that the connecting line of both poles will always pass through the affected part (muscle or joint). At the same time the brush is to be rapidly lifted, and in the same rapid manner placed upon an adjoining portion, so that gradually (about within a period of one to two minutes) the skin situated over the inflamed place appears to be moderately reddened. General electrization and electrical baths are also well recommended, especially in the chronic stage. The same treatment will be found useful in other inflammations of the joints, in rheumatic contractions, and also in both atrophy and hypertrophy of the muscles.

Spasms of the face. Tic convulsif. Treatment: Faradic brushing of the skin of the neck and mastoid process (situated behind the ear) for ten minutes.

Spinal Meningitis—Inflammation of the membranes of the spinal marrow. Myelitis—Inflammation of the spinal marrow.

Electrical treatment has been successful only in the chronic stage.

Treatment: General Faradisation and the Faradic brush applied to the back and extremities.

Tabes dorsalis, spinal paralysis, induration of the spinal marrow are to be treated by the application, (repeated once a week) of the Faradic brush to the skin of the entire body (the head excepted). Faradisation with a weak current has also been of use if applied in the following manner: the negative pole placed upon the neck close to the angle of the lower maxillary (jaw) bone, while the positive pole with the moist roller attached thereto, is passed slowly downwards on the opposite side of the cervical column, closely along the spinous processes, beginning with an even pressure, at the shoulder blades. The roller is then repassed upwards in a somewhat quicker and easier manner, and then passed down again as before. After three to four minutes the same manipulation is repeated on the opposite side. It will be of great advantage to combine the electrical with such other general treatment as may be indicated by the general symptoms. We take this occasion to refer, in general to the essay "Pulmonary Consumption," consumption phthisis pulmonum. We deem it impossible to treat this widely spread, dangerous affection, exclusively with the electrical current. The influence of the electrical current upon the tubercular degeneration of the lungs, or, if any body is ready to take it for granted, upon the cause of this affection, "the bacillus tuberculosus" has not yet been sufficiently investigated to take a new departure and provide a new and, at the same time, efficient treatment against it. The writer of this essay having for many years thoroughly investigated and practically treated this affection, has ascertained that the cause of eighty per cent. of cases of pulmonary consumption can be traced to a mechanical disturbance of the bony frame work and, especially to curvature of the spine and mal position of the chest. Hence an unwholesome pressure is brought to bear upon the heart, lungs, stomach, etc. Respiration, circulation of the blood, and also the nutrition of the entire body gradually becomes more defective, until finally all the symptoms occur which are characteristic of pulmonary consumption. Unless the cause of the disease is removed, which means in this case the mal position of the bony frame, which, in our opinion, can only be accomplished, in a satisfactory manner according to mechanical principles, we must consider a complete cure rather problematical. Those interested in this theory are referred to the author's pamphlet about the "Health Restoring Belt," invented by him. The electrical treatment, however, has been in many cases of great value, especially as a stimulant to the accessory nerves, the dorsalis scapulae, levator scapulae, cucullaris, the anterior thoracic nerves, the thoracicus longus, vagus and sympatheticus, also of the external intercostal muscles, opisthothenar, etc. For this purpose the Faradic brush and the moist electrode will be found useful as a tonic for the muscles of the chest, by passing it over the entire thorax in a lateral direction and from above downwards. Application of the brush may also be made to the costal border in order to cause a salutary action upon the liver, spleen and kidneys. It is our intention to write a special essay on the influence of electricity in the treatment and cure of pulmonary consumption.

The two affections, *struma* (goître) and *scrophula* (infiltration of the glands) may be reduced and even obliterated by daily Faradisation of from eight to ten minutes length of time. Both electrodes are placed upon the tumor in such a manner that the action of the current acts upon it in the largest possible circumference. The treatment frequently demands both time and patience.

Ulcus, ulcer. See erysipelas. There is still another series of morbid symptoms which can be successfully treated with electricity, and specially through Faradisation. The number of these diseases steadily increases in proportion to the spreading of the use of electricity as a remedial agent. If the principle is maintained, that electricity is one of the most preferable agents for restoring and stimulating the various organs of the body, into renewed normal action, and thus enablling them to overcome morbid conditions, to destroy and expel deleterious substances, it must seem natural that general affections will, by means of general electrization and electrical baths, be influenced in a favorable manner. The same may be said concerning the electrical treatment in local affections (disease of the liver, kidneys, spleen, biliousness, etc.,) by a suitable and merely local application of the electrical current to the corresponding parts of the body. It would exceed the space allowed for this purpose to enumerate every single morbid symptom, but the remarks therefore made and the annexed drawings together with the index will enable most any one to treat, if necessary, such as are not mentioned in this essay. Thus the use of electricity in the treatment of disease will gradually become general property.

To assist in this work and to bring about its accomplishment is the intention of this essay.

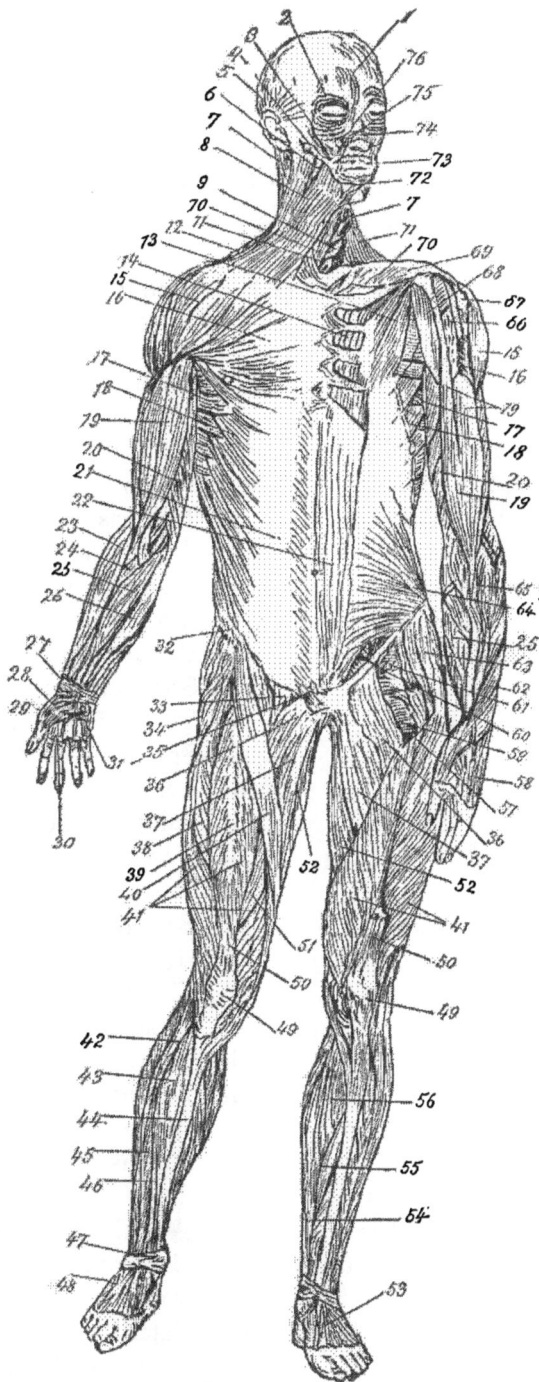

FIGURE 2.

MUSCULAR SYSTEM OF MAN.

FRONT VIEW. FIG. 2.

The superficial muscles of the neck, shoulder, forearm and thigh
are partially off.

1. Frontal portion of the Occipito-Frontalis
2. Orbicularis Palpebrarum
3. Zygomaticus Minor
4. " Major
5. Temporal
6. Buccinator
7. Sterno-Mastoideus
8. Digastricus
9. Thyroid Gland
10. Sterno-Hyoid
11. Trachea
12. Cucullaris
13. Pectoralis Minor
14. Intercostal
15. Deltoid
16. Pectoralis Major
17. Serratus Magnus anticus
18. Obliquus Externus
19. Biceps
20. Triceps
21. Sheath of Tendon of Rectus Muscle
22. Rectus Muscle
23. Brachialis Anticus
24. Pronator Radii Teres
25. Flexor Sublimis Digitorum
26. Internal Muscle of the Elbow

27. Anterior Common Ligament of the Wrist Joint
28. Abductor Brevis Pollicis
29. Flexor Brevis Pollicis
30. Tendons of the Flexor Digit
31. Musculus Palmaris Brevis
32. Crest of the Ileum
33. Spsoas magnus
34. Tensor fasciae latae
35. Spermatic cord
36. Pectoneus
37. Adductor Longus
38. Vastus Externus
39. Rectus
40. Sartorius
41. Gastrocnemius
42. Tibialis
43. Tibialis Anticus
44. Shin bone
45. Extensor Longus Digitorum
46. Extensor Proprius Pollicis
47. Annular Ligament
48. Extensor Brevis Digitorum
49. Patella
50. Extensor Tendon

51. Vastus Externus Muscle
52. Gracilio sive Rectus internus
53. Extensor Tendons of the Toes
54. Tendo Achilles
55. Flexor Longus Digitorum
56. Tibialis Posticus
57. Poupart's Ligament
58. Tendon of Extensor Muscle
59. Obturator Externus Muscle
60. Inguinal Canal Muscle
61. Head of Femur "
62. Abductor Pollicis "
63. Gluteus Medius "
64. Obliquus Internus Abdom Muscle

65. Flexor Sublimus Digit Muscle
66. Long Tendon of the Biceps Muscle
67. Head of the upper Arm
68. Coracco Brachialis M.
69. Clavide
70. Sub-clavian Muscle
71. Scalenus "
72. Depressor of the lower Lip
73. Sphinctre Muscle of the Mouth.
74. Compressor of the Nose
75. Levator of the upper Lip and of the wing of the Nose
76. Levator of the upper Lip

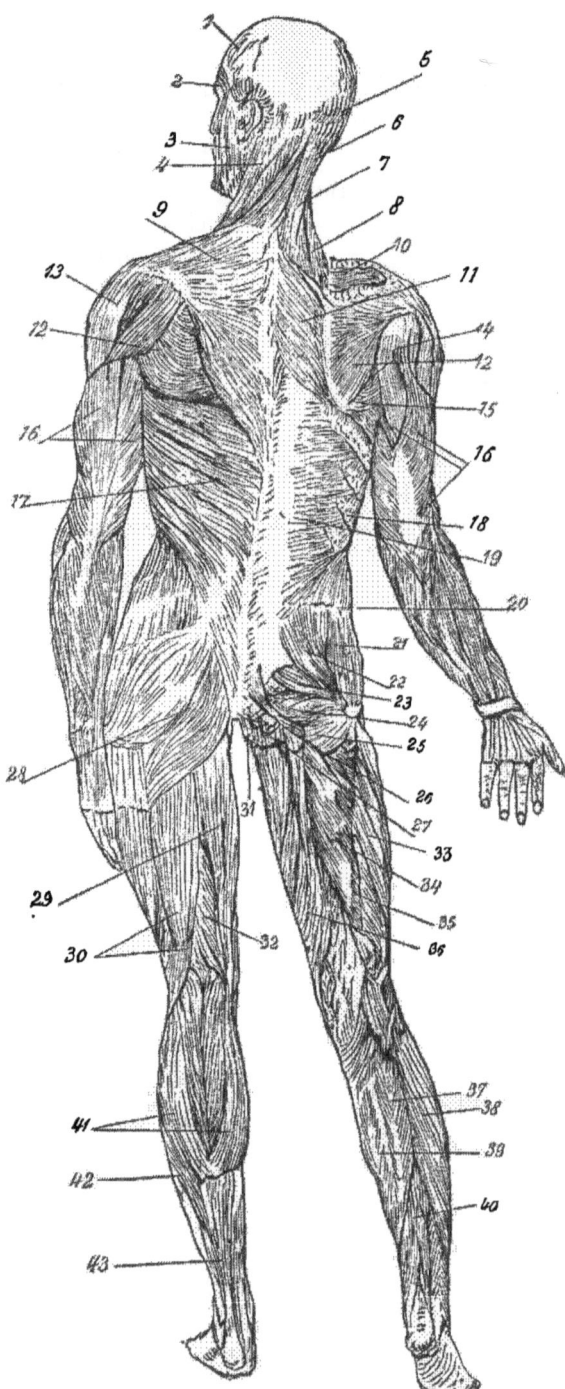

FIGURE 3.

MUSCULAR SYSTEM OF MAN.

BACK VIEW. FIG. 3.

1. Frontalis
2. Sphincter of the eyelid
3. Masseter
4. Sternocleido-mastoideus
5. Occipitalis
6. Splenius capitis
7. " colli
8. Levator anguli
9. Cucullaris
10. Supraspinatus
11. Rhomboideus
12. Infraspinatus
13. Deltoideus
14. Teres minor
15. Teres major
16. Triceps
17. Latissimus dorsi
18. Ribs
19. Inferior posticus seratus
20. Crest of the ileum
21. Glutaeus medius
22. " parvus
23. Pyriformis

24. Obturator internus
25. Quadratus femoris
26. Ligamentum tuberosa-crum
27. Os coccygis
28. Glutaeus maximus
29. Gracilis
30. Biceps femoris
31. Tuber ischii
32. Semi-tendinosus
33. Vastus externus
34. Adductor magnus femoris
35. Femur
36. Semi-membranosus
37. Tibialis posticus
38. Peroneus
39. Extensor digitorum communis longus
40. Extensor hallucis longus
41. Gastrocnemius
42. Soleus
43. Tendo Achillis

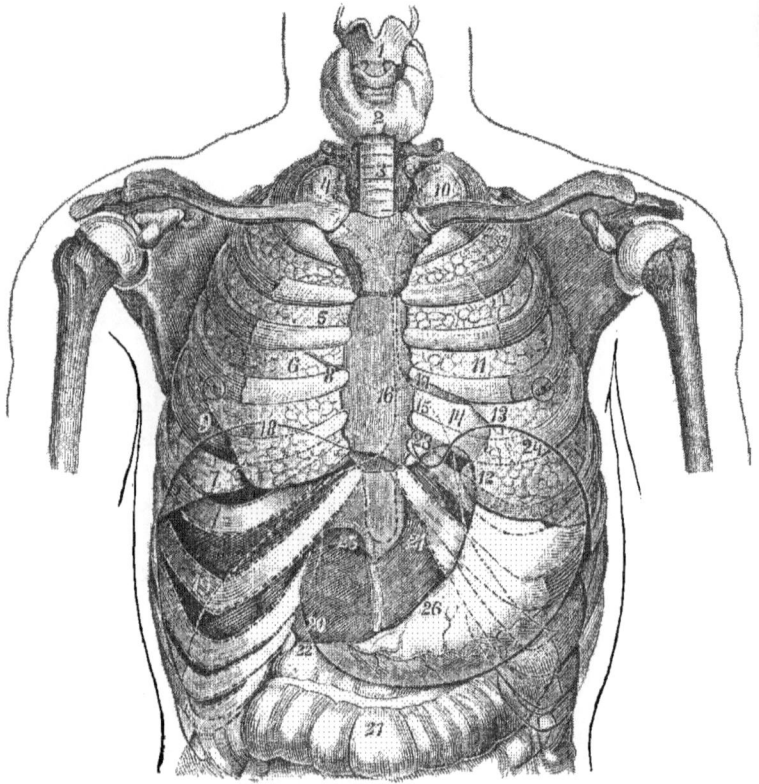

FIGURE 4.

FIG. 4. ANTERIOR VIEW OF THE THORACIC AND

ABDOMINAL ORGANS.

1. Larynx
2. Thyroid gland
3. Trachea
4. Top (apex) of right lung
5. Upper lobe   "   "
6. Median "   "   "
7. Lower "   "   "
8. Upper incisura (cleft) interlobularis
9. Lower incisura (cleft) interlobularis
10. Apex (top)
11. Upper lobe of the left lung
12. Lingual process of the upper lobe of the left lung.
13. Cardiae incision of the anterior margin of the left lung.
14. Front side of the pericardium, partially covered by the cardiac pleura

15. The same not covered by the pleura
16. Upper border of the right mediastinum
17. Anterior border of the left mediastinum
18. Upper border of the liver, partially covered by the right lung.
19. Right lobe of the liver
20. Quadrangular lobe of the liver
21. Left lobe of liver.
22. Gall bladder
23. Upper opening of the stomach
24. Fundus of the stomach, partially covered by the lung.
25. Pylorus
26. Greater curvature
27. Transverse colon

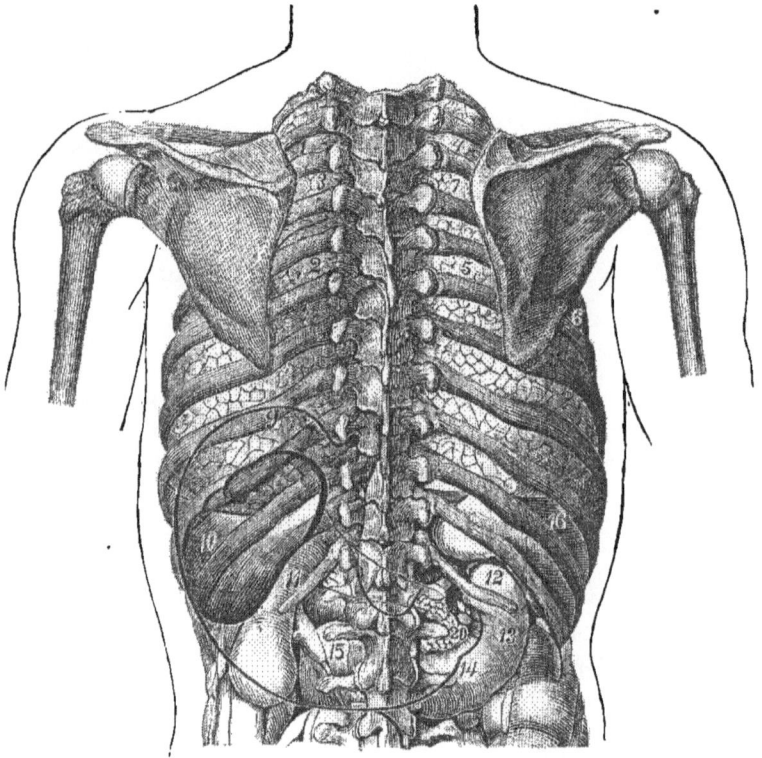

FIGURE 5.

Fig. 5.   Posterior view of the Organs situated within the Chest and Abdomen.

1. Upper lobe of the left lung
2. Lower lobe of the left lung
3. Interlobular groove of the left lung.
4. Upper lobe of the right lung
5. Lower lobe of the right lung
6. Middle lobe of the right lung
7. Superior groove of the right lung
9. The stomach, with a dark outline
10. The spleen, drawn in its relation to: the lungs during expiration and, to the kidney during expiration.
11. Left kidney
12. Horizontal portion of the upper duodenum
13. Descending portion of the same.
14. Horizontal portion of the duodenum
15. Flexura duodeno-jejunaeis
16. Liver.
17. Pancreas

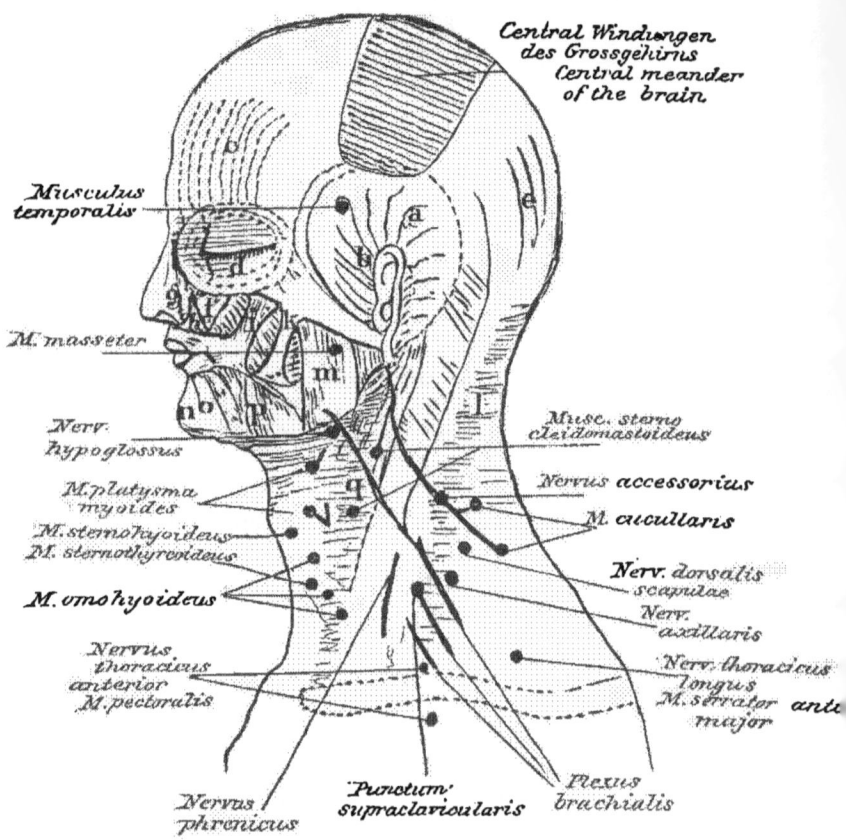

Central Windungen
des Grossgehirns
Central meander
of the brain

Musculus temporalis

M. masseter

Nerv. hypoglossus

M. platysma myoides
M. sternohyoideus
M. sternothyroideus

M. omohyoideus

Nervus thoracicus anterior
M. pectoralis

Nervus phrenicus

Punctum supraclavicularis

Musc. sterno cleidomastoideus

Nervus accessorius
M. cucullaris

Nerv. dorsalis scapulae
Nerv. axillaris

Nerv. thoracicus longus
M. serrator ante major

Plexus brachialis

FIGURE 6.

a. Attolens jauriculae muscle
b. Temporal muscle
c. Frontal portion of occipito-frontalis muscle
d. Orbicularis palpebrarum muscle
e. Occipital portion of occipito-frontalis muscle
f. Levator labii superioris muscle
g. Levator labii superioris alaeque nasi muscle
h. Sterno-cleido-mastoidens muscle

i. Zygomaticus minor muscle
k.   "   major   "
l. Cucullaris muscle
m. Masseter   "
n. Levator menti muscle
o. Depressor labii inferioris muscle
p. Depressor anguli oris muscle
q. Platysma myoides, sive subcutaneous colli
Central meander, sive convolutions of the main brain.

SCHEDULE OF NERVES AND MUSCLE.
HEAD AND NECK.

Effect of electrical irritation upon the nerve and muscle.

Facial nerve—Distortion of the entire face to the corresponding side.

Posterior auricular nerve—Contraction of the posterior occipital muscles of the levator and retractor of the ear, in consequence of which also elevation of the ear upwards and backwards.

Accessory nerve—Bending of the spinal column and simultaneous rotation of the head around its axis towards the opposite side, protusion of the lower jaw bone, elevation of the shoulders.

Dorsal nerve of the shoulder blade—Contraction of the rhomboideus and serratus posticus superior. Elevation of the shoulder blade towards the cervical column and slight elevation of the upper ribs.

Phrenic nerve—Contraction of the diaphragm, protrusion of the abdomen with hiccough, a sudden rush of air into the windpipe.

Anterior thoracic nerves—Contraction of the larger and smaller pectoral muscles and adduction of the arm to the interior surface of the trunk.

Hypoglossus nerve—Elevation of the tongue.

Frontal muscle—Wrinkling of the brow in a horizontal direction and distortion of the frontal portion and upper eyelids.

Temporal muscle—Powerful closing of the lower jaw.

Corrugator of the eye lid—Irritation of both eyes is followed by vertical contraction of the forehead unilateral, but pulling down of the eyebrows.

Orbicularis palpebrae—Closing of the eyes, corrugation of the eyelids.

Levator of the wing of the nose and upper lip—Elevation of the upper lip and wing of the nose, next corrugation of the. nose.

Compressor of the nose—Pulling of the eyebrows inwards and downwards.

Splenius capitis et collis—Turning of the head towards the point of irritation.

Sternocleido-mastoideus—Turning of the head towards the opposite side, bending of the cervical column forwards. Faradisation of both sides moves the head with a strong curvature of the cervical column, elevation of the chin forwards.

Zygomatic major et minor—For the greater zygomatic muscle, elevation of the angle of the mouth and of the upper lip, corrugation of the cheek. For the zygomatic minor, raising of the upper lip upwards and outwards. Protrusion and constriction of the lips.

Orbicularis oris—Protrusion and contraction of the lips.

Masseter—The same as in the temporal muscle.

Levator menti—Flattening of the chin and displacement of the lower lip.

Depressor labii inferioris—Pulling down of the lower lip and pressing of the same against the teeth.

Depressor anguli oris—Pulling down and drawing outwards of the angle of the mouth and of the lower lip and, consequently, enlargement of aperture of the mouth.

Levator of the scapula—Elevation of the shoulder-blade, especially of its internal angle upwards and forwards.

Cucullaris—Elevation of the shoulder and drawing down of the head posterially.

Platysma myoides of the hyodean bones—

Omohyoideus—

Axillary nerve—Contraction of the deltoid muscle.

Thoracicus longus nerve—Motion of the shoulder-blade forwards and outwards. The collar bone is lifted off the chest, causing a deepening of the clavicular grooves.

Plesus brachialis—Motion of the entire arm. The supraclavicular point, also, belongs to this plexus.

ON THE TRUNK.

Intercostales externi—Elevation of the rib situated next to the electrode.

Rectus abdominis—Flattening of the abdominal convexity.

Transversus abdominis—Contraction of the abdominal muscles.

Obliquus abdominis—In bilateral stimulation, lateral flattening and median elevation of the abdominal wall.

Latissimus dorsi—Is to be stimulated from the corresponding nerve.

Serratus posticus inferior—Can be directly stimulated.

Teres major—Can be directly stimulated.

Externor dorsi communis—Spinal column bends in the corresponding direction, the other spinal roots cannot be stimulated.

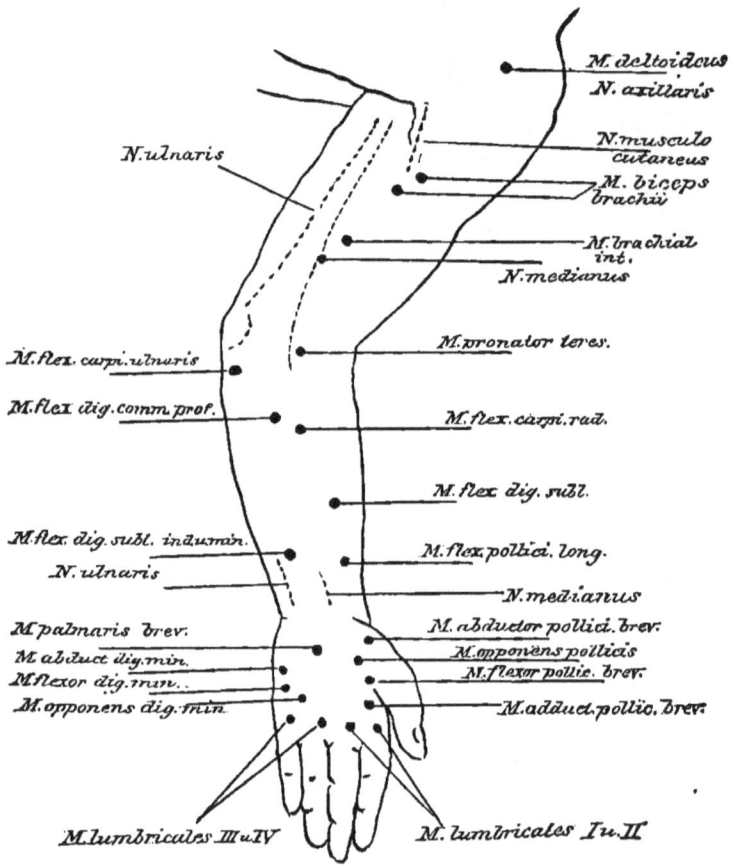

M. deltoideus
N. axillaris

N. musculo cutaneus
M. biceps brachii

M. brachial int.
N. medianus

M. pronator teres.

N. ulnaris

M. flex. carpi. ulnaris

M. flex. dig. comm. prof.

M. flex. carpi. rad.

M. flex. dig. subl.

M. flex. dig. subl. induman.
N. ulnaris

M. flex. pollici. long.

N. medianus

M. palmaris brev.
M. abduct. dig. min.
M. flexor dig. min.
M. opponens dig. min.

M. abductor pollici. brev.
M. opponens pollicis
M. flexor pollic. brev.
M. adduct. pollic. brev.

M. lumbricales III u. IV

M. lumbricales I u. II

FIGURE 7.

MUSCLES OF THE ARM. FIG. 7.

Deltoid—
Triceps—
Biceps—
Nervus cutaneous brachii externus, or Nervus musculocutaneous—
 Contraction of the biceps, flexion of the forearm.
Brachialis internus—
*Nervus ulnaris—*Contraction of the inner muscles of the
 elbow, of the common deep flexor of the fingers, of the
 palmaris brevis, etc., causing the hand to be contracted.
*Nervus medianus—*Vigorous turning of the forearm inwards
 and flexion of the fingers.
Supinator longus, or brachio-radialis—
Pronator teres—
Flexor carpi ulnaris—
  " *digitorum communis profundus—*
  " *carpi radialis—*
  " *digit. communis sublimis—*
  " *pollicis longus—*
Nervus medianus—
  " *ulnaris—*
Abductor pollicis brevis—
Opponeus pollicis—
Flexor pollicis brevis—
Abductor "   " —
Palmaris brevis—
Abductor digiti minimi—
Flexor brevis digiti minimi—
Oppeneus "   " —
Musculi lumbricales—

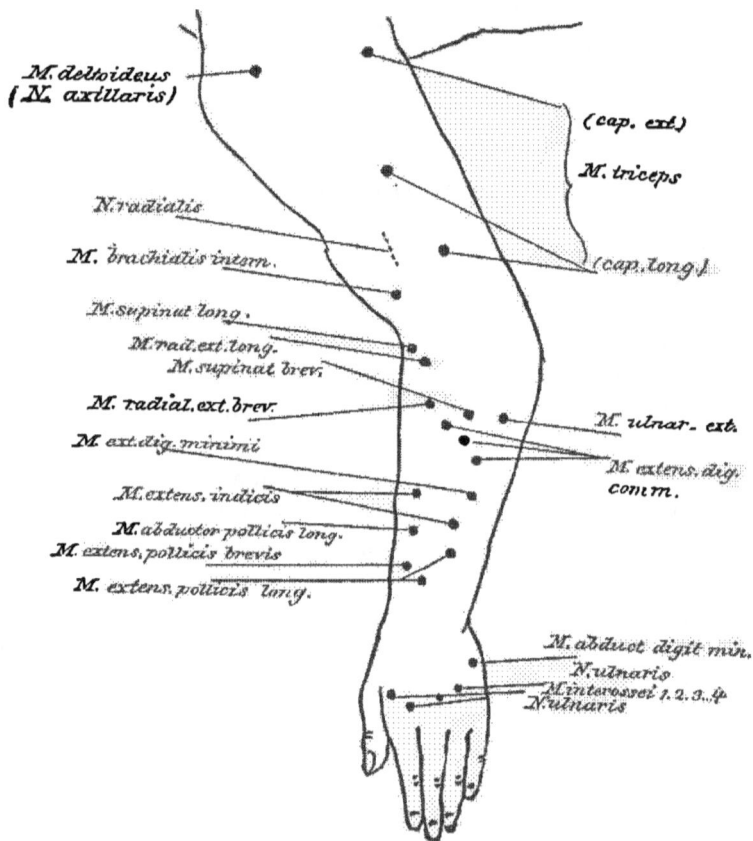

M. deltoideus
(N. axillaris)

(cap. ext.)

M. triceps

N. radialis

M. brachialis intern.

(cap. long.)

M. supinat long.

M. rad. ext. long.
M. supinat brev.

M. radial. ext. brev.

M. ext. dig. minimi

M. ulnar. ext.

M. extens. dig.
comm.

M. extens. indicis

M. abductor pollicis long.
M. extens. pollicis brevis

M. extens. pollicis long.

M. abduct digit min.
N. ulnaris
M. interossei 1. 2. 3.. 4
N. ulnaris

FIGURE 8.

Figure 8.

Deltoideus—
Triceps caput longum—
    "   "   *esternum—*

*N. radialis—*Contraction of a larger group of muscles, turning of the forearm outwards with extension of the hand, thumb and first digital bone.

Brachialis internus—
Supinator longus—
Radialis externor longus—
    "   "   *brevis—*
Extensor digitorum communis—
Supinator brevis—
Ulnaris externus—
Extensor digiti minimi—
    "   *indicis—*
Abductor pollicis longus —
Extensor   "   brevis—
Abductor digiti minimi—
Interossei externi—

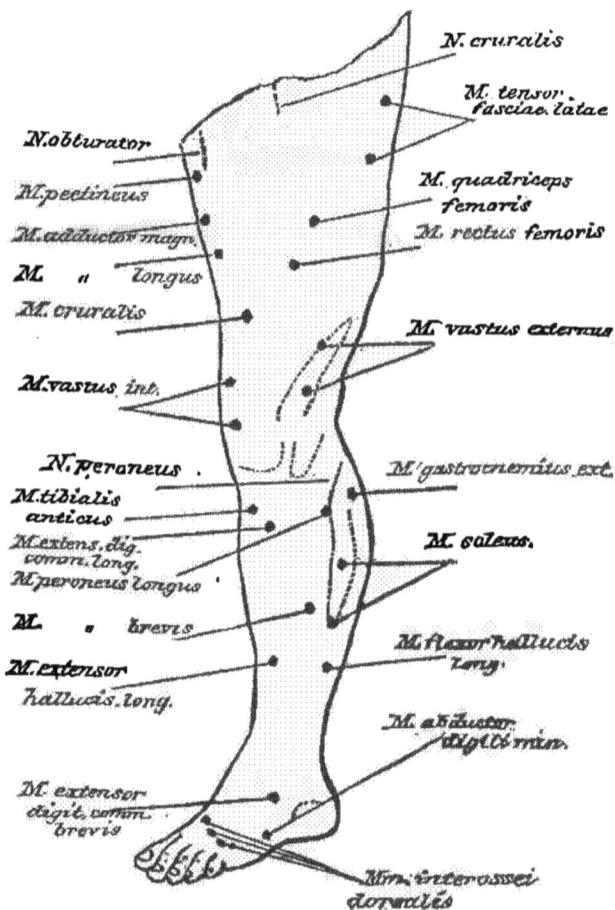

N. cruralis

M. tensor
fasciae latae

N. obturator

M. pectineus

M. adductor magn.

M. quadriceps
femoris

M. rectus femoris

M. " longus

M. cruralis

M. vastus externus

M. vastus int.

N. peroneus

M. gastrocnemius ext.

M. tibialis
anticus

M. extens. dig.
comm. long.

M. soleus.

M. peroneus longus

M. " brevis

M. extensor
hallucis. long.

M. flexor hallucis
long.

M. abductor
digiti min.

M. extensor
digit. comm.
brevis

Mm. interossei
dorsales

FIGURE 9.

LEGS.   FIG. 9.

Nervus cruralis—Extension of the leg.
Musc. tensor fascinlatae—
N. obturatorius—Powerful adduction of the thigh.
Pectineus—
Sartorius—
Abductor magnus—
    " *longus—*
Extensor quadriceps—
Femoris—
Rectus femoris
Cruralis—
Vastus externus—
    " *internus—*
Tibialis anticus—
Extensor digit. com. longus—
Peroneus brevis—
Extensor haltucis longus—
Interossei pedis—
Extensor digitorum communis brevis—
Abductor digit. min.—
Peroneus longus—

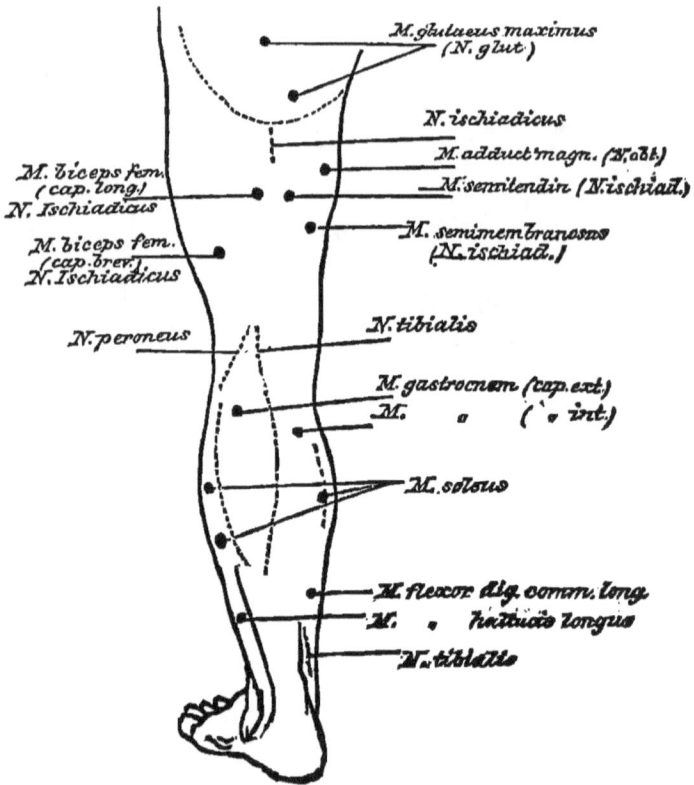

FIGURE 10.

Glutaeus maximus—

*N. ischiadicus—*Flexion of the leg, contraction of all the
muscles belonging to the leg and foot.

Abductor magnus—

Semitendinosus—

Biceps femoris—

N. Tibialis—Contraction of all the muscles of the posterior surface and of the sole of the foot.

Peroneus—

Gastrocnemius—

Soleus

Flexor digitorum pedis communis—

    "   *hallucis longus—*

www.ingramcontent.com/pod-product-compliance
Lightning Source LLC
Chambersburg PA
CBHW032123080426
42733CB00008B/1034